Dash Diet Cookbook For Your Lunch

A perfect mix of Tasty Recipes to stay healthy and fit or to enjoy your everyday Lunch Meals

Natalie Puckett

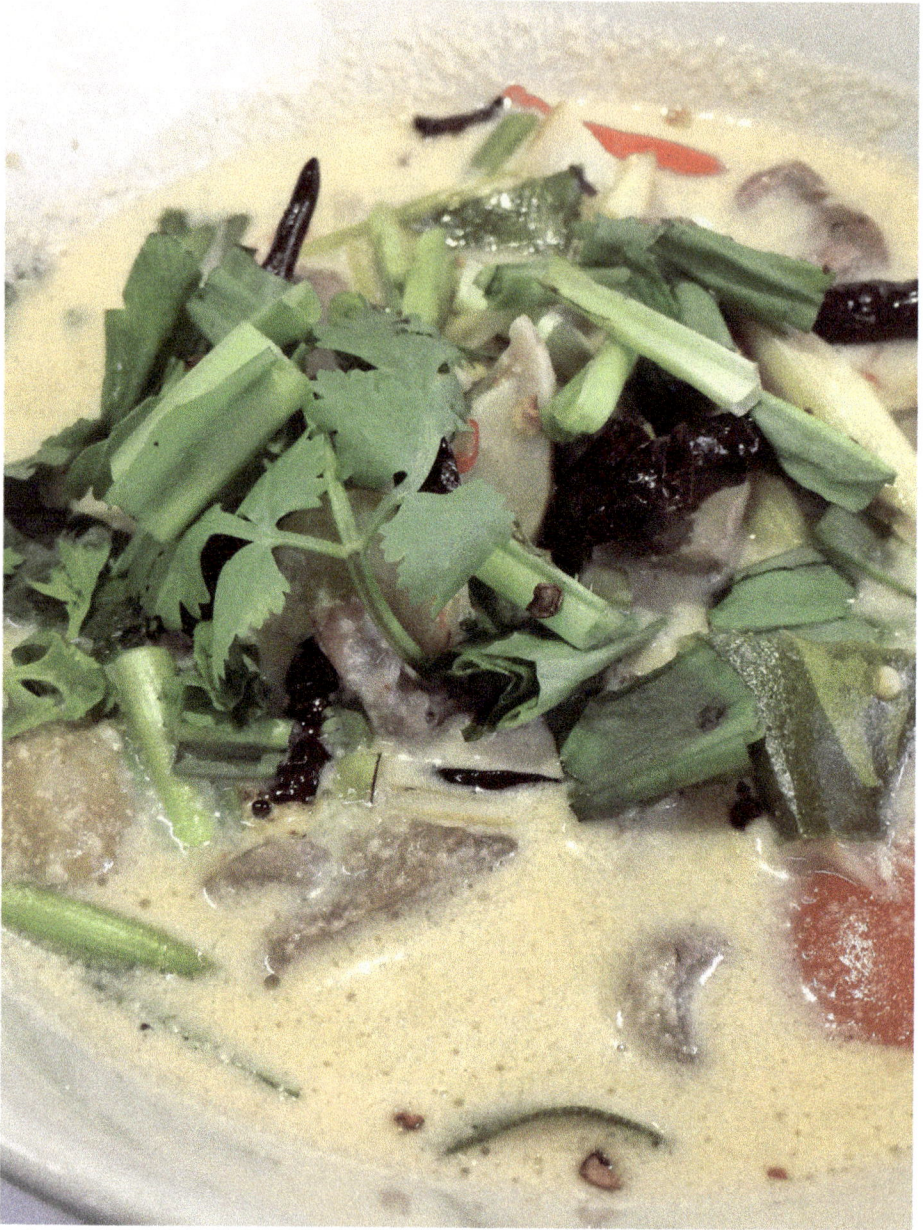

Table of Contents

COCONUT ARUGULA SOUP 5

AWESOME CABBAGE SOUP 7

BAKED ZUCCHINI WRAPPED FISH 9

HEART-WARMING MEDI TILAPIA 12

BAKED SALMON AND ORANGE JUICE 14

LEMON AND ALMOND BUTTER COD... 16

SHRIMP SCAMPI...18

LIGHT BEEF CHILI 20

INSALATA GRECA 24

CRUDITIES .... .26

SIMPLE GINGERBREAD MUFFINS 27

FANTASTIC CAULIFLOWER BAGELS 29

NUTMEG NOUGATS 31

LIMEY SAVORY PIE 33

SUPREME RASPBERRY CHOCOLATE BOMBS 35

THE PERFECT ORANGE PONZU 37

HEARTY CASHEW AND ALMOND BUTTER................................... 40

REFRESHING MANGO AND PEAR SMOOTHIE 42

EPIC PINEAPPLE JUICE 44

CHOCO LOVERS STRAWBERRY SHAKE 47

HEALTHY COFFEE SMOOTHIE 49

BLACKBERRY AND APPLE SMOOTHIE...50

LEMONY SPROUTS 51

COOL GARBANZO AND SPINACH BEANS 53

ITALIAN TURKEY SAUSAGE AND VEGETABLE OMELET 55

CHINESE-STYLE ZUCCHINI WITH GINGER 57

BREAKFAST SUPER ANTIOXIDANT BERRY SMOOTHIE 60

CUCUMBER TOMATO SURPRISE...62

AVOCADO NORI ROLLS 64

Maple Ginger Pancakes 66

Chewy Chocolate Chip Cookies 68

Lovely Faux Mac and Cheese 70

Epic Mango Chicken 73

Chicken and Cabbage Platter 75

Hearty Chicken Liver Stew 77

Chicken Quesadilla 79

Zucchini Beef Sauté with Coriander Greens 81

Hearty Lemon and Pepper Chicken 83

Walnuts and Asparagus Delight 86

Healthy Carrot Chips 88

Garden Vegetable and Herb Soup 90

Salad Chard and White Bean Pasta 92

Cauliflower with Roasted Almond and Pepper Dip 94

Spicy Grilled Broccoli 96

Super-easy Chicken Noodle Soup 99

Hearty Ginger Soup 102

Tasty Tofu and Mushroom Soup 104

Ingenious Eggplant Soup 106

Loving Cauliflower Soup 108

Coconut Arugula Soup

Serving: 4

Prep Time: 5 minutes

Cook Time: 5-10 minutes

Ingredients:

Black pepper as needed

1 tablespoon olive oil

2 tablespoons chives, chopped

2 garlic cloves, minced

10 ounces baby arugula

2 tablespoons tarragon, chopped

4 tablespoons coconut milk yogurt

6 cups chicken stock

2 tablespoons mint, chopped

1 onion, chopped

½ cup coconut milk

How To:

1.   Take a saucepan and place it over medium-high heat, add oil and let it heat up.

2.   Add onion and garlic and fry for five minutes.

3.   Stir available and reduce the warmth, let it simmer.

4.   Stir in tarragon, arugula, mint, parsley and cook for six minutes.

5.   Mix in seasoning, chives, coconut yogurt and serve.

6.   Enjoy!

Nutrition (Per Serving)

Calories: 180

Fat: 14g

Net Carbohydrates: 20g

Protein: 2g

Awesome Cabbage Soup

Serving: 3

Prep Time: 7 minutes

Cook Time: 25 minutes

Ingredients:

3 cups non-fat beef stock

2 garlic cloves, minced

1 tablespoon tomato paste

2 cups cabbage, chopped

½ yellow onion

½ cup carrot, chopped

½ cup green beans

½ cup zucchini, chopped

½ teaspoon basil

½ teaspoon oregano

Sunflower seeds and pepper as needed

How To:

1.   Grease a pot with non-stick cooking spray.

2.   Place it over medium heat and permit the oil to heat up.

3.   Add onions, carrots, and garlic and sauté for five minutes.

4.   Add broth, ingredient, green beans, cabbage, basil, oregano, sunflower seeds, and pepper.

5.   Bring the entire mix to a boil and reduce the warmth, simmer for 5-10 minutes until all veggies are tender.

6.   Add zucchini and simmer for five minutes more.

7.   Sever hot and enjoy!

Nutrition (Per Serving)

Calories: 22

Fat: 0g

Carbohydrates: 5g

Protein: 1g

Baked Zucchini Wrapped Fish

Serving: 2

Prep Time: 15 minutes

Cook Time: 15 minutes

Ingredients:

24-ounce cod fillets, skin removed

tablespoon of blackening spices

zucchini, sliced lengthwise to form ribbon

½ tablespoon of olive oil

How To:

1.   Season the fish fillets with blackening spice.

2.   Wrap each fillet with zucchini ribbons.

3.   Place fish on a plate.

4.   Take a skillet and place over medium heat.

5.   Pour oil and permit the oil to heat up.

6.   Add wrapped fish to the skillet and cook all sides for 4 minutes.

7.   Serve and enjoy!

Nutrition (Per Serving)

Calories: 397

Fat: 23g

Carbohydrates: 2g

Protein: 46g

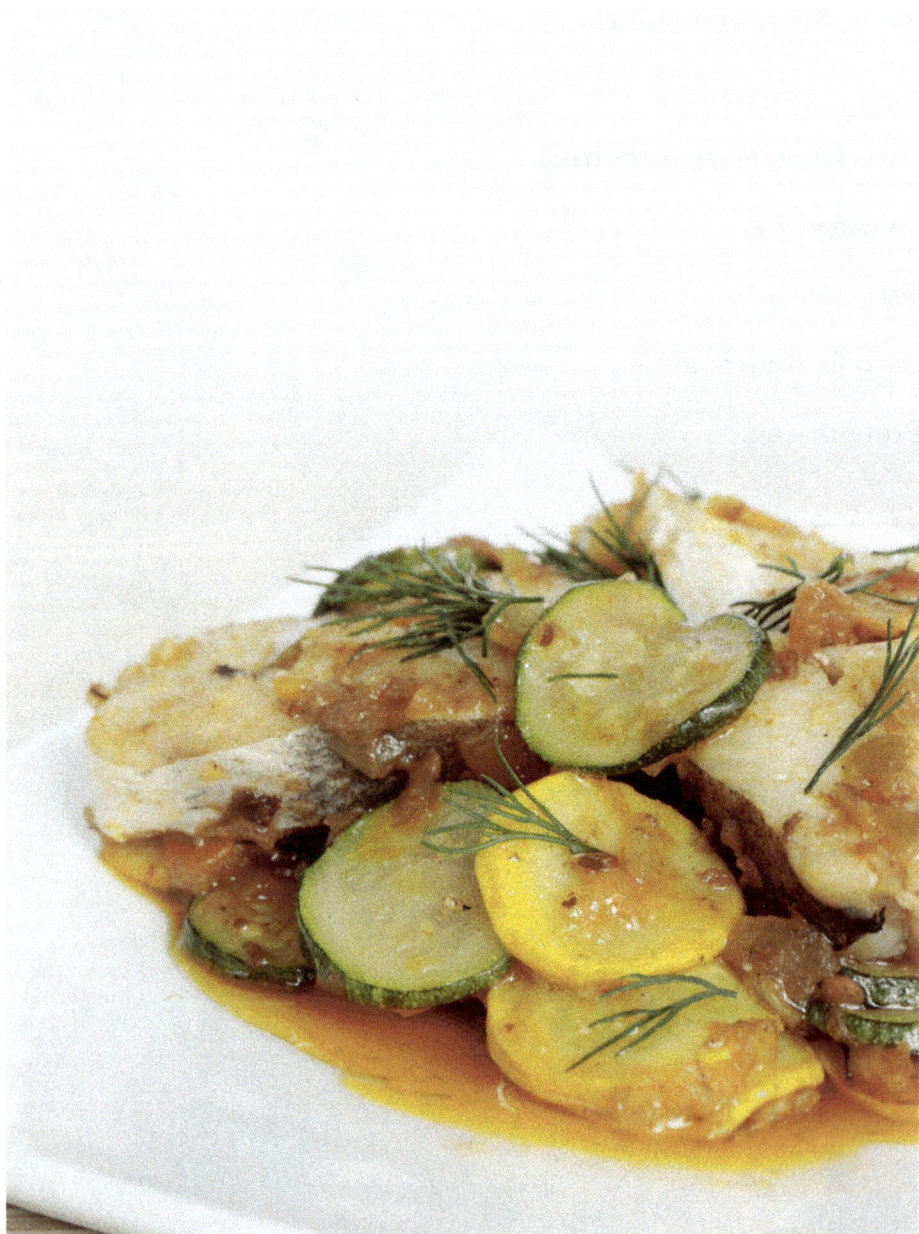

Heart-Warming Medi Tilapia

Serving: 4

Prep Time: 15 minutes

Cook Time: 15 minutes

Ingredients:

tablespoons sun-dried tomatoes, packed in oil, drained and chopped

tablespoon capers, drained

tilapia fillets

tablespoon oil from sun-dried tomatoes tablespoons kalamata olives, chopped and pitted

How To:

1.   Pre-heat your oven to 372 degrees F.

2.   Take alittle sized bowl and add sun-dried tomatoes, olives, capers and stir well.

3.   Keep the mixture on the side.

4.   Take a baking sheet and transfer the tilapia fillets and arrange them side by side.

5.   Drizzle vegetable oil everywhere them.

6.   Bake in your oven for 10-15 minutes.

7.   After 10 minutes, check the fish for a "Flaky" texture.

8.   Once cooked, top the fish with the tomato mixture and serve!

Nutrition (Per Serving)

Calories: 183

Fat: 8g

Carbohydrates: 18g

Protein:83g

Baked Salmon and Orange Juice

Serving: 2

Prep Time: 10 minutes

Cook Time: 10 minutes

Ingredients:

½ pound salmon steak

Juice of 1 orange

Pinch ginger powder, black pepper, and sunflower seeds

Juice of ½ lemon

1-ounce coconut almond milk

How To:

1.   Preheat oven to 350 degrees F.

2.   Rub salmon steak with spices and let it sit for quarter-hour.

3.   Take a bowl and squeeze an orange.

4.   Squeeze juice also and blend.

5.   Pour almond milk into the mixture and stir.

6.   Take a baking dish and line with aluminium foil .

7.   Place steak thereon and pour the sauce over steak.

8.   Cover with another sheet and bake for 10 minutes.

9.   Serve and enjoy!

Nutrition (Per Serving)

Calories: 300

Fat: 3g

Carbohydrates: 1g

Protein: 7g

Lemon and Almond butter Cod

Serving: 2

Prep Time: 5 minutes

Cook Time: 20 minutes

Ingredients:

tablespoons almond butter, divided thyme sprigs, fresh and divided teaspoons lemon juice, fresh and divided

cod fillets, 6 ounces each Sunflower seeds to taste

How To:

1.   Pre-heat your oven to 400 degrees F.

2.   Season cod fillets with sunflower seeds on each side.

3.   Take four pieces of foil, each foil should be 3 times bigger than the fillets.

4.   Divide fillets between the foil and top with almond butter, juice, thyme.

5.   Fold to make a pouch and transfer pouches to the baking sheet.

6.   Bake for 20 minutes.

7.   Open and let the steam out.

8.   Serve and enjoy!

Nutrition (Per Serving)

Calories: 284

Fat: 18g

Carbohydrates: 2g

Protein: 32g

Shrimp Scampi

Serving: 4

Prep Time: 25 minutes

Cook Time: Nil

Ingredients:

teaspoons olive oil

1 ¼ pounds medium shrimp

6-8 garlic cloves, minced

½ cup low sodium chicken broth

½ cup dry white wine

¼ cup fresh lemon juice

¼ cup fresh parsley + 1 tablespoon extra, minced ¼ teaspoon sunflower seeds

¼ teaspoon fresh ground pepper

slices lemon

How To:

1.   Take an outsized sized bowl and place it over medium-high heat.

2.   Add oil and permit the oil to heat up.

3.   Add shrimp and cook for 2-3 minutes.

4.   Add garlic and cook for 30 seconds.

5.   Take a slotted spoon and transfer the cooked shrimp to a serving platter.

6.   Add broth, juice, wine, ¼ cup of parsley, pepper, and sunflower seeds to the skillet.

7.   Bring the entire mix to a boil.

8.   Keep boiling until the sauce has been reduced to half.

9.   Spoon the sauce over the cooked shrimp.

10.   Garnish with parsley and lemon.

11.   Serve and enjoy!

Nutrition (Per Serving)

Calories: 184
Fat: 6g
Carbohydrates: 6g
Protein: 15g

Light Beef Chili

SmartPoints value: Green plan - 4SP, Blue plan - 4SP, Purple plan – 4SP

Total Time: 2hrs 30mins, Prep time: 30mins, Cooking time: 2hrs, Serves: 8

Nutritional value: Calories - 187, Carbs – 24g, Fat – 3g, Protein – 16g

Ingredients

Beef bouillon powder - 1 tbsp

Bell pepper (red, diced) - 1 small

Black pepper - 1/2 tsp

Brewed coffee (strong) - 1 cup

Chili powder - 3 tbsp

Cocoa (unsweetened) - 1 tsp

Cumin - 2 tbsp

Dark beer - One 12oz can

Garlic (minced) - 4 cloves

Green pepper (diced) - 1 small

Ground beef (extra lean) - 1 lb

Kidney beans - One 15oz can

Onion (diced) - 1 large

Oregano - 2 tsp

Paprika - 1 tsp

Salt - 1 tsp

Sugar - 1 tbsp

Tomatoes (diced) - One 28oz can

Tomato sauce - One 8oz can

Instructions

1.   Place a large pot or Dutch oven over medium-high heat and spray it with non-fat cooking spray.

2.   Add the onions and garlic, then cook until onions start to soften; about 3 minutes.

3.   Toss in the ground beef and cook until the meat turns brown.

4.   Add the diced bell peppers to the beef and cook for another 5 minutes.

5.   Put in all the remaining ingredients asides the kidney beans and stir.

6.   Bring the content of the pot to a simmer, then stir in the kidney beans.

7.   Reduce the heat to medium-low, cover the pot, and let it cook for about 2 hours.

This perfect hearty beef chili made with extra lean ground beef simmers in fantastic spices and flavors to give you a desirable taste.

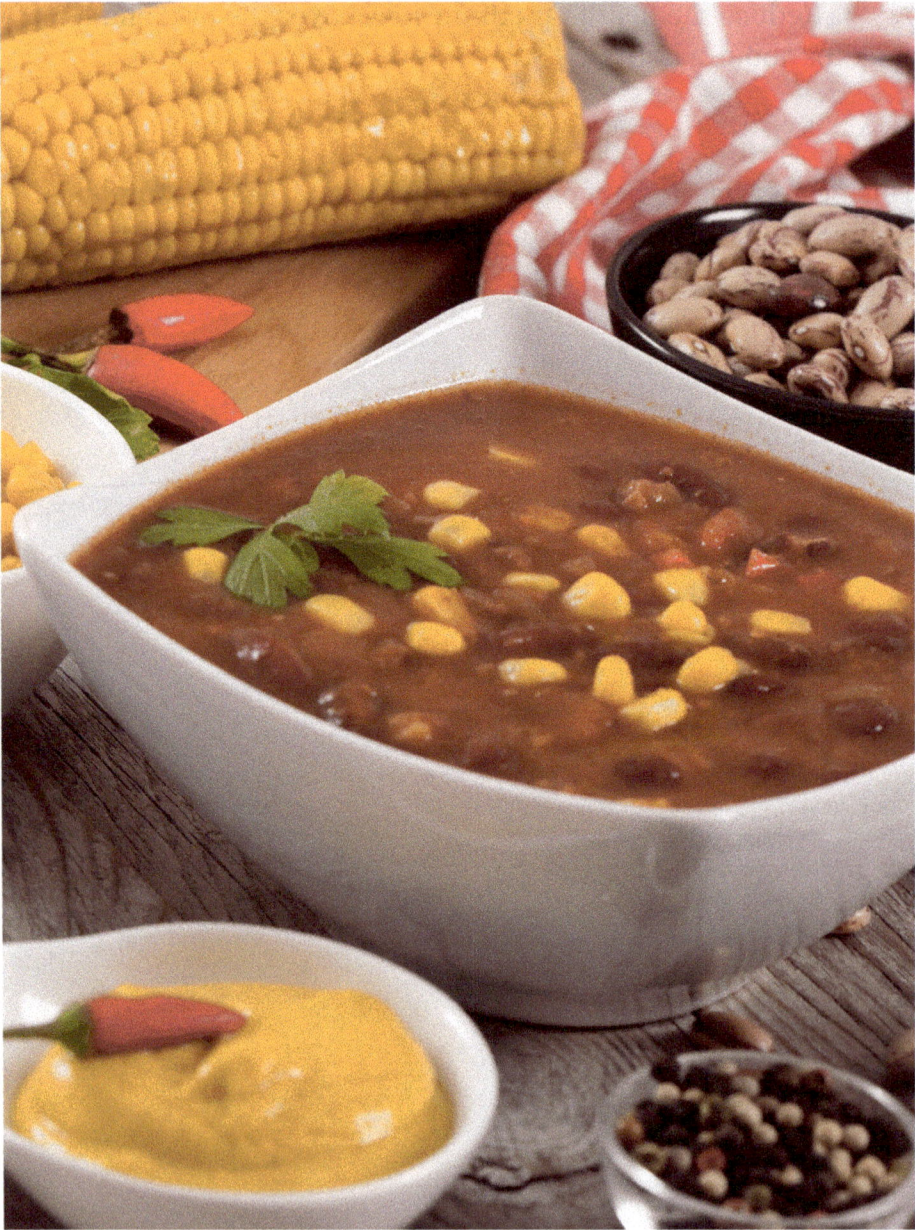

Insalata Greca

Nutrition

Calories: 326 kcal | Gross carbohydrates: 11 g | Protein: 14 g | Fats: 26 g |

Fiber: 4 g | Net carbohydrates: 7 g | Macro fats: 55 % | Macro proteins: 30 % |

Macro carbohydrates: 15 %

Total time: 5 minutes

Ingredients

50 grams of tomato

50 grams of cucumber

25 grams of red pepper or yellow pepper

15 grams of red onion

50 grams of feta

50 grams of black olives

3 tablespoons extra virgin olive oil

1 tablespoon lemon juice

1 teaspoon dried oregano

1 egg

Instructions

1.   Bring a saucepan of water to the boil. Once the water boils, place the egg in it. Boil the egg for 8 minutes.

2.   Clean the onion and cut into thin slices (keep the rest of the onion in a sealed container in the refrigerator).

3.   Wash the tomato, pepper, and cucumber and cut the pepper and cucumber into thin slices. Dice the tomato.

4.   Peel the egg and cut it into slices.

5.   Arrange the tomatoes and the egg in the center of a plate. Put the cucumber slices around it. Place the bell pepper and red onion on top of the tomatoes.

6.   Drain the feta if necessary and cut into small 1 cm large cubes. Place in a heap on top of the tomato.

7.   Decorate the dish with the black olives and sprinkle the oregano over the tomatoes.

8.   Make the vinaigrette in a small cup or bowl by mixing the olive oil and lemon juice well with a fork or teaspoon.

9.   Pour the vinaigrette over the salad.

Crudities

Total time: 10 minutes

Ingredients

1 celery stem

1 bush of chicory cuts lengthwise into four pieces Cut 10 cm cucumber into long, thin strips

2 peppers, for example, red and yellow

Instructions

1.   Cut the vegetables into thin, long strips so that you can dip them. For example, you can use chicory, little gem lettuce, cucumber, colored peppers, and celery.

2.   Tasty and fast - if you don't feel like cooking.

Nutrition

Calories: 22 kcal | Gross carbohydrates: 5 g | Protein: 1 g | Fats: 0.2 g | Fiber: 2 g | Net carbohydrates: 3 g | Macro fat: 5 % | Macro proteins: 24 % | Macro carbohydrates: 71 %

Simple Gingerbread Muffins

Serving: 12

Prep Time: 5 minutes

Cooking Time: 30 minutes

Ingredients:

1 tablespoon ground flaxseed

6 tablespoons coconut almond milk

1 tablespoon apple cider vinegar

½ cup peanut almond butter

2 tablespoons gingerbread spice blend

1 teaspoon baking powder

1 teaspoon vanilla extract

2 tablespoons Swerve

How To:

1.   Pre-heat your oven to 350 degrees F.

2.   Take a bowl and add flaxseeds, sweetener, sunflower seeds, vanilla, spices and your non-dairy almond milk.

3.   Keep it on the side for a while.

4.   Add peanut almond butter, baking powder and keep mixing until combined well.

5.   Stir in peanut almond butter and baking powder.

6.   Mix well.

7.   Spoon the mixture into muffin liners.

8.   Bake for 30 minutes.

9.   Allow them to cool and enjoy!

Nutrition (Per Serving)

Total Carbs: 13g

Fiber: 4g

Protein: 11g

Fat: 23g

Fantastic Cauliflower Bagels

Serving: 12

Prep Time: 10 minutes

Cooking Time: 30 minutes

Ingredients:

1 large cauliflower, divided into florets and roughly chopped

¼ cup nutritional yeast

¼ cup almond flour

½ teaspoon garlic powder

1 ½ teaspoon fine sea sunflower seeds

1 whole egg

1 tablespoon sesame seeds

How To:

1.   Pre-heat your oven to 400 degrees F.

2.   Line a baking sheet with parchment paper, keep it on the side.

3.   Blend cauliflower in the food processor and transfer to a bowl.

4.   Add nutritional yeast, almond flour, garlic powder and sunflower seeds to a bowl, mix.

5.   Take another bowl and whisk in eggs, add to cauliflower mix.

6.   Give the dough a stir.

7.   Incorporate the mix into the egg mix.

8.   Make balls from dough, making a hole using your thumb into each ball.

9.   Arrange them on your prepped sheet, flattening them into bagel shapes.

10.   Sprinkle sesame seeds and bake for 30 minutes.

11.   Remove oven and let them cool, enjoy!

Nutrition (Per Serving)

Total Carbs: 1.5g

Fiber: 1g

Protein: 2g

Fat: 5.8g

Nutmeg Nougats

Serving: 12

Prep Time: 10 minutes

Cooking Time: 5 minutes

Freeze Time: 30 minutes

Ingredients:

1 cup coconut, shredded

1 cup low-fat cream

1 cup cashew almond butter

½ teaspoon ground nutmeg

How To:

1. Melt the cashew almond butter over a double boiler.

2. Stir in nutmeg and dairy cream.

3. Remove from the heat.

4. Allow to cool down a little.

5. Keep in the refrigerator for at least 30 minutes.

6.   Take out from the fridge and make small balls.

7.   Coat with shredded coconut.

8.   Let it cool for 2 hours and then serve.

Nutrition (Per Serving)

Total Carbs: 13g

Fiber: 8g

Protein: 3g

Fat: 34g

Limey Savory Pie

Serving: 12

Prep Time: 5 minutes

Cooking Time: 5 minutes

Freeze Time: 2 hours

Ingredients:

1 tablespoon ground cinnamon

3 tablespoons almond butter

1 cup almond flour

For the filling:

3 tablespoons grass-fed almond butter

4 ounces full-fat cream cheese

¼ cup coconut oil

2 limes

A handful of baby spinach Stevia to taste

How To:

1.　　Mix cinnamon and almond butter to form a crumble mixture.

2.　　Press this mixture into the bottom of 12 muffin cups.

3.　　Bake for 7 minutes at 350 degrees F.

4.　　Juice the lime and grate for zest while the crust is baking.

5.　　Take a food processor and add all the filling ingredients.

6.　　Blend until smooth.

7.　　Let it cool naturally.

8.　　Pour the mixture in the center.

9.　　Freeze until set and serve.

Nutrition (Per Serving)

Total Carbs: 2g

Fiber: 1g

Protein: 3g

Fat: 1g

Supreme Raspberry Chocolate Bombs

Serving: 6

Prep Time: 10 minutes

Cooking Time: 10 minutes

Freeze Time: 1-hour

Ingredients:

½ cacao almond butter

½ coconut manna

4 tablespoons powdered coconut almond milk

3 tablespoons granulated stevia

¼ cup dried and crushed raspberries, frozen

How To:

1.   Prepare your double boiler to medium heat and melt the cacao almond butter and coconut manna.

2.   Stir in vanilla extract.

3.   Take another dish and add coconut powder and sugar substitute.

4.   Stir the coconut mix into the cacao almond butter, 1 tablespoon at a time, making sure to keep mixing after each addition.

5.   Add the crushed dried raspberries.

6.   Mix well and portion it out into muffin tins.

7.   Chill for 60 minutes and enjoy!

Nutrition (Per Serving)

Total Carbs: 7g

Fiber: 1g

Protein: 11g

Fat: 21g

The Perfect Orange Ponzu

Serving: 8

Prep Time: 30 minutes

Cook Time: 5 minutes

Ingredients:

¼ cup coconut aminos

½ cup rice vinegar

2 tablespoons dry fish flakes

1 (1 inch) square kombu (kelp)

1 orange, quartered

How To:

1.   Take a saucepan and place it over medium heat.

2.   Add coconut aminos, rice vinegar, fish flakes, kombu, orange quarters and let the mixture sit for 30 minutes.

3.   Bring the mix to a boil and immediately remove from the heat.

4.   Let it cool and strain through a cheesecloth.

5.	Serve and enjoy!

Nutrition (Per Serving)

Calories: 15

Fat: 0g

Carbohydrates: 4g

Protein: 0.8g

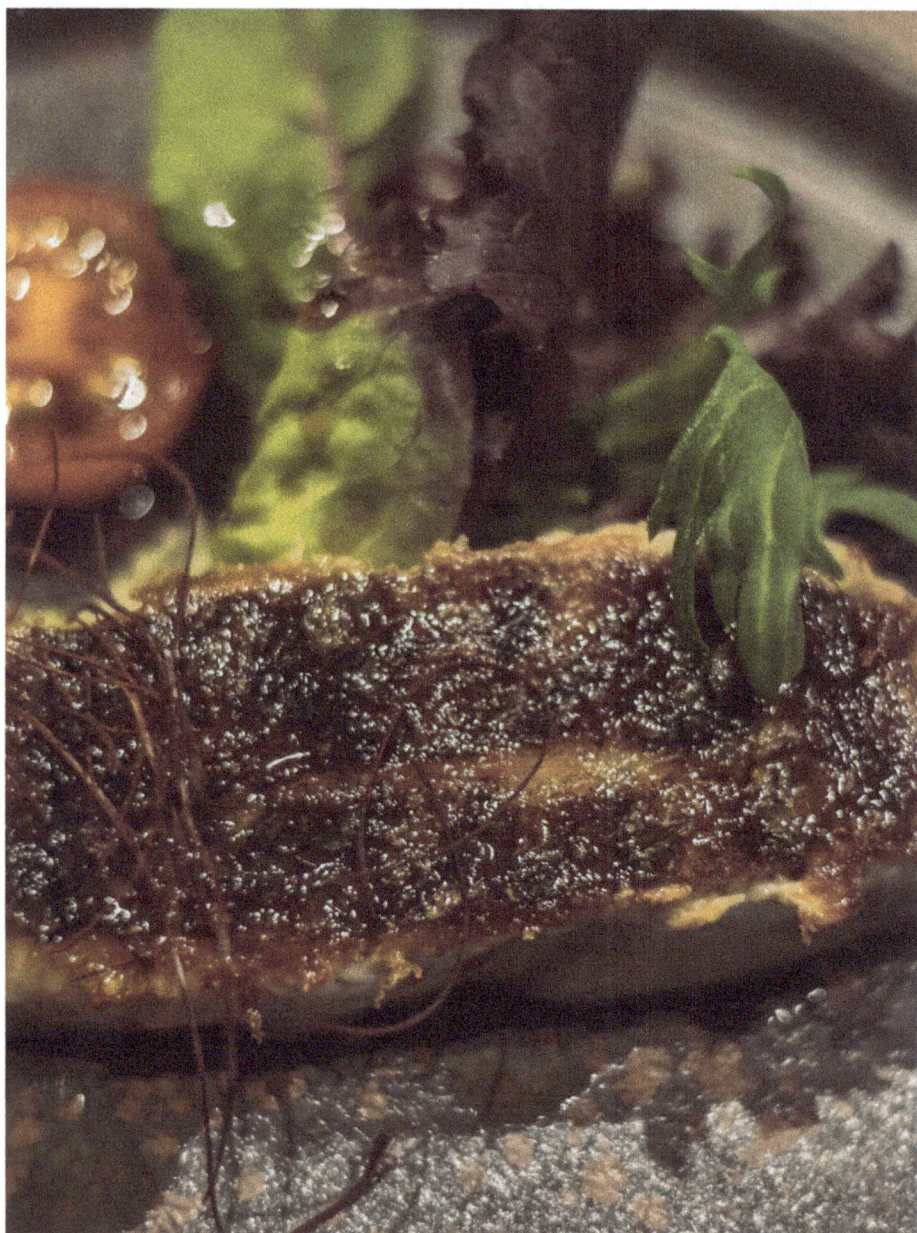

Hearty Cashew and Almond butter

Serving: 1 and ½ cups

Prep Time: 5 minutes

Cook Time: Nil

Ingredients:

1 cup almonds, blanched

1/3 cup cashew nuts

2 tablespoons coconut oil

Sunflower seeds as needed

½ teaspoon cinnamon

How To:

1.   Pre-heat your oven to 350 degrees F.

2.   Bake almonds and cashews for 12 minutes.

3.   Let them cool.

4.   Transfer to food processor and add remaining ingredients.

5.   Add oil and keep blending until smooth.

6.   Serve and enjoy!

Nutrition (Per Serving)

Calories: 205

Fat: 19g

Carbohydrates: g[MOU3]

Protein: 2.8g

Refreshing Mango and Pear Smoothie

Serving: 1

Prep Time: 10 minutes

Cook Time: Nil

Ingredients:

1 ripe mango, cored and chopped

½ mango, peeled, pitted and chopped

1 cup kale, chopped

½ cup plain Greek yogurt

2 ice cubes

How To:

1.   Add pear, mango, yogurt, kale, and mango to a blender and puree.

2.   Add ice and blend until you have a smooth texture.

3.   Serve and enjoy!

Nutrition (Per Serving)

Calories: 293

Fat: 8g

Carbohydrates: 53g

Protein: 8g

Epic Pineapple Juice

Serving: 4

Prep Time: 10 minutes

Cook Time: nil

Ingredients:

4 cups fresh pineapple, chopped

1 pinch sunflower seeds

1 ½ cups water

How To:

1.   Add the listed ingredients to your blender and blend well until you have a smoothie-like texture.

2.   Chill and serve.

3.   Enjoy!

Nutrition (Per Serving)

Calories: 82

Fat: 0.2g

Carbohydrates: 21g

Protein: 21

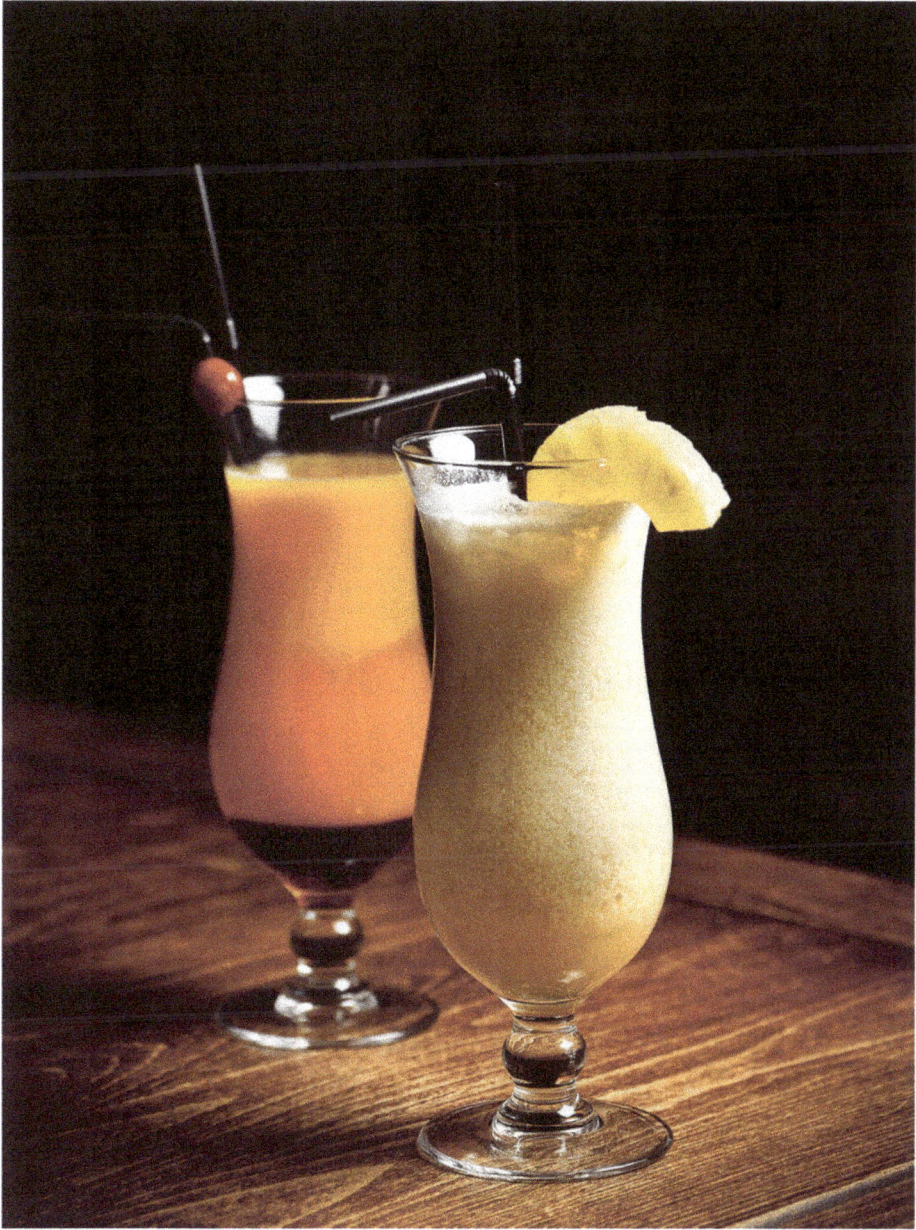

Choco Lovers Strawberry Shake

Serving: 1

Prep Time: 10 minutes

Ingredients:

½ cup heavy cream, liquid

1 tablespoon cocoa powder

1 pack stevia

½ cup strawberry, sliced

1 tablespoon coconut flakes, unsweetened

1 ½ cups water

How To:

1. Add listed ingredients to blender.

2. Blend until you have a smooth and creamy texture.

3. Serve chilled and enjoy!

Nutrition (Per Serving)

Calories: 470

Fat: 46g

Carbohydrates: 15g

Protein: 4g

Healthy Coffee Smoothie

Serving: 1

Prep Time: 10 minutes

Ingredients:

1 tablespoon chia seeds

2 cups strongly brewed coffee, chilled

1-ounce Macadamia Nuts

1-2 packets stevia, optional

1 tablespoon MCT oil

How To:

1.   Add all the listed ingredients to a blender.

2.   Blend on high until smooth and creamy.

3.   Enjoy your smoothie.

Nutrition (Per Serving)

Calories: 395

Fat: 39g

Carbohydrates: 11g

Protein: 5.2g

Blackberry and Apple Smoothie

Serving: 2

Prep Time: 5 minutes

Ingredients:

2 cups frozen blackberries

½ cup apple cider

1 apple, cubed

2/3 cup non-fat lemon yogurt

How To:

1.   Add the listed ingredients to your blender and blend until smooth.

2.   Serve chilled!

Nutrition (Per Serving)

Calories: 200
Fat: 10g
Carbohydrates: 14g
Protein 2g

Lemony Sprouts

Serving: 4

Prep Time: 10 minutes

Cook Time: Nil

Ingredients:

1 pound Brussels sprouts, trimmed and shredded

8 tablespoons olive oil

1 lemon, juice and zested

Sunflower seeds and pepper to taste

¾ cup spicy almond and seed mix

How To:

1. Take a bowl and mix in lemon juice, sunflower seeds, pepper and olive oil.

2. Mix well.

3. Stir in shredded Brussels sprouts and toss.

4. Let it sit for 10 minutes.

5.   Add nuts and toss.

6.   Serve and enjoy!

Nutrition (Per Serving)

Calories: 382

Fat: 36g

Carbohydrates: 9g

Protein: 7g

Cool Garbanzo and Spinach Beans

Serving: 4

Prep Time: 5-10 minutes

Cook Time: Nil

Ingredients:

1 tablespoon olive oil

½ onion, diced

10 ounces spinach, chopped

12 ounces garbanzo beans

½ teaspoon cumin

How To:

1.   Take a skillet and add olive oil, let it warm over medium-low heat.

2.   Add onions, garbanzo and cook for 5 minutes.

3.   Stir in spinach, cumin, garbanzo beans and season with sunflower seeds.

4.   Use a spoon to smash gently.

5.   Cook thoroughly until heated, enjoy!

Nutrition (Per Serving)

Calories: 90

Fat: 4g

Carbohydrates:11g

Protein:4g

Italian Turkey Sausage and Vegetable Omelet

Ingredients

Cooked chicken or turkey sausage(s) - 1½ oz, Italian-variety, chopped

Fresh edible mushroom(s) - ¾ cup(s), chopped

Fresh parsley - ½ Tbsp, chopped

Uncooked onion(s) - ¼ cup(s), chopped

Cooking spray - 4 spray(s)

Egg(s) - 2 large, beaten with a pinch of salt and pepper

Grated Pecorino Romano cheese - 1½ Tbsp

Chopped and roasted red peppers (packed in water) - ¼ cup(s)

Instructions

1.   Coat a small-sized omelet pan with cooking spray and heat over medium flame.

2.   Add the sausage, mushroom, and onion, then cook, frequently stirring, until the onions soften, 5 minutes. Remove the cooked omelet from pan to a bowl and stir in roasted pepper, then set aside.

3.   Wipe the pan clean with a paper towel.

4.   Put off heat, coat the pan again with cooking spray, and heat over medium flame.

5.   Add the beaten eggs and swirl to spread egg over the pan.

6.   Cook it until the bottom is done and the top is nearly cooked for about 3 minutes.

7.   Top the omelet with chicken sausage mixture and sprinkle with cheese.

8.   Fold the omelet over and cook for 1-2 minutes more. Serve it sprinkled with parsley.

Chinese-Style Zucchini with Ginger

Servings per container - 10

Prep Total - 10 min

Serving Size 2/3 cup (55g)

Nutritional Facts

Total Fat 8g

Total Carbohydrate 37g

Protein 3g

Sodium 160mg

Ingredients:

1 teaspoon oil

1 lb. zucchini cut into 1/4-inch slices

1/2 cup vegetarian broth

2 teaspoon light soy sauce

1 teaspoon dry sherry

1 teaspoon toasted sesame oil

Instructions:

1.   Heat a large wok or heavy skillets over high heat until very hot then add the oil. When the oil is hot, add the zucchini and ginger.

2.   Stir-fry 1 minute.

3.   Add the broth, soy sauce, and sherry.

4.   Stir-fry over high heat until the broth cooks down a bit and the zucchini is crisp-tender.

5.   Remove from the heat, sprinkle with sesame oil and serve.

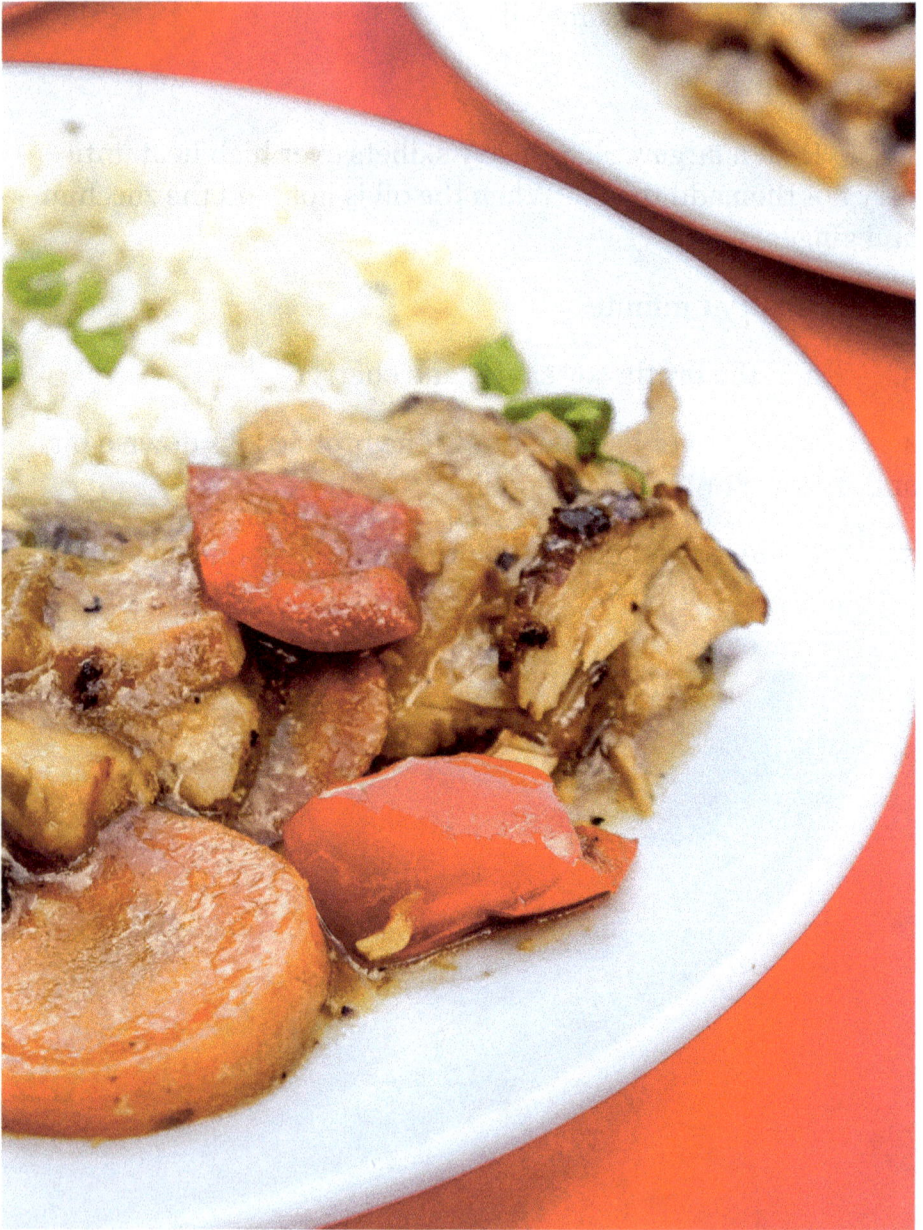

Breakfast Super Antioxidant Berry Smoothie

servings per container - 5

Prep Total - 10 min

Serving Size - 4 cup (20g)

Nutritional Facts

Total Fat 2g

Sodium 7mg

Total Carbohydrate 20g

Protein 3g

Ingredients

1 cup of filtered water

1 whole orange, peeled, de-seeded & cut into chunks

2 cups frozen raspberries or blackberries

1 Tablespoon goji berries

1 1/2 Tablespoons hemp seeds or plant-based protein powder

2 cups leafy greens (parsley, spinach, or kale)

Instructions:

Blend on high until smooth

Serve and drink immediately

Cucumber Tomato Surprise

servings per container - 5

Prep Total - 10 min

Serving Size 2/3 cup (55g)

Nutritional Facts

Total Fat 20g

Total Carbohydrate 14g

Total Sugar 2g

Protein 7g

Ingredients

Chopped 1 medium of tomato

1 small cucumber peeled in stripes and chopped

1 large avocado cut into cubes

1 half of a lemon or lime squeezed

1/21 tsp. Himalayan or Real salt

1 Teaspoon of original olive oil, MCT or coconut oil

Instructions:

1.   Mix everything together and enjoy

2.   This dish tastes even better after sitting for 40 – 60 minutes

3.   Blend into a soup if desired.

Avocado Nori Rolls

Nutritional Facts

servings per container	10
Prep Total	**10 min**
Serving Size 2/3 cup (70g)	
Amount per serving **Calories**	**15**
	% Daily Value
Total Fat 2g	**10%**
Saturated Fat 1g	9%
Trans Fat 10g	-
Cholesterol	**1%**
Sodium 70mg	**5%**
Total Carbohydrate 22g	**40%**
Dietary Fiber 4g	2%
Total Sugar 12g	-
Protein 3g	
Vitamin C 2mcg	2%
Calcium 260mg	7%
Iron 8mg	2%
Potassium 235mg	4%

Ingredients

2 sheets of raw or toasted sushi nori

1 large Romaine leaf cut in half down the length of the spine

2 Teaspoon of spicy miso paste

1 avocado, peeled and sliced

½ red, yellow or orange bell pepper, julienned

½ cucumber, peeled, seeded and julienned

½ cup raw sauerkraut

½ carrot, beet or zucchini, shredded

1 cup alfalfa or favorite green sprouts

1 small bowl of water for sealing roll

Instructions:

1.   Place a sheet of nori on a sushi rolling mat or washcloth, lining it up at the end closest to you.

2.   Place the Romaine leaf on the edge of the nori with the spine closest to you.

3.   Spread Spicy Miso Paste on the Romaine

4.   Line the leaf with all ingredients in descending order, placing sprouts on last

5.   Roll the Nori sheet away from you, tucking the ingredients in with your fingers, and seal the roll with water or Spicy Miso Paste. Slice the roll into 6 or 8 rounds.

Maple Ginger Pancakes

Nutritional Facts

servings per container	4
Prep Total	**10 min**
Serving Size 2/3 cup (20g)	
Amount per serving **Calories**	**20**
	% Daily Value
Total Facts 10g	**10%**
Saturated Fat 0g	7%
Trans **Fat** 2g	-
Cholesterol	**3%**
Sodium 10mg	**2%**
Total Carbohydrate 7g	**3%**
Dietary Fiber 2g	4%
Total Sugar 1g	-
Protein 3g	
Vitamin C 2mcg	10%
Calcium 260mg	20%
Iron 8mg	30%
Potassium 235mg	6%

Ingredients

1 or 2 cup flour

1 tablespoonful baking powder

1/2 tablespoonful kosher salt

1/4 tablespoonful ground ginger

1/4 table spoonful pumpkin pie spice

1/3 cup maple syrup

2/4 cup water

minced 1/4 cup + 1 tablespoonful crystallized ginger slices together

Instructions:

1.   In a neat bowl mix together the first five recipes

2.   Add flour with syrup with water and stir together, after that add in the chopped ginger & stir until-just-combined.

3.   Heat your frying pan and coat with a nonstick cooking spray

4.   Pour in 1/4 cup of the batter and allow to heat until it forms bubbles. Allow to cook until browned

5.   Serve warm & topped with a slathering of vegan butter, a splash of maple syrup, and garnished with chopped candied ginger.

Chewy Chocolate Chip Cookies

Nutritional Facts

servings per container	10
Prep Total	**10 min**
Serving Size 2/3 cup (40g)	
Amount per serving **Calories**	**10**
	% Daily Value
Total Fat 10g	**2%**
Saturated Fat 1g	5%
Trans Fat 0g	-
Cholesterol	**15%**
Sodium 120mg	**8%**
Total Carbohydrate 21g	**10%**
Dietary Fiber 4g	1%
Total Sugar 1g	0%
Protein 6g	
Vitamin C 2mcg	7%
Calcium 210mg	51%
Iron 8mg	1%
Potassium 235mg	10%

Ingredients

1 cup vegan butter, softened

½ cup white sugar

½ cup brown sugar

¼ cup dairy-free milk

1 teaspoon vanilla

2 ¼ cups flour

½ teaspoon salt

1 teaspoon baking soda

12 ounces dairy-free chocolate chips

Instructions:

1.   Preheat oven to 350°F.

2.   In a large bowl, mix the butter, white sugar, and brown sugar until light and fluffy. Slowly stir in the dairy-free milk and then add the vanilla to make a creamy mixture.

3.   In a separate bowl, combine the flour, salt, and baking soda.

4.   You need to add this dry mixture to the liquid mixture and stir well. Fold in the chocolate chips.

5.   Drop small spoonful of the batter onto non-stick cookie sheets and bake for 9 minutes.

Lovely Faux Mac and Cheese

Serving: 4

Prep Time: 15 minutes

Cook Time: 45 minutes

Ingredients:

5 cups cauliflower florets

Sunflower seeds and pepper to taste

1 cup coconut almond milk

½ cup vegetable broth

2 tablespoons coconut flour, sifted

1 organic egg, beaten

1 cup cashew cheese

How To:

1.   Preheat your oven to 350 degrees F.

2.   Season florets with sunflower seeds and steam until firm.

3.   Place florets during a greased ovenproof dish.

4. Heat coconut almond milk over medium heat during a skillet, confirm to season the oil with sunflower seeds and pepper.

5. Stir in broth and add coconut flour to the combination, stir.

6. Cook until the sauce begins to bubble.

7. Remove heat and add beaten egg.

8. Pour the thick sauce over the cauliflower and blend in cheese.

9. Bake for 30-45 minutes.

10. Serve and enjoy!

Nutrition (Per Serving)

Calories: 229

Fat: 14g

Carbohydrates: 9g

Protein: 15g

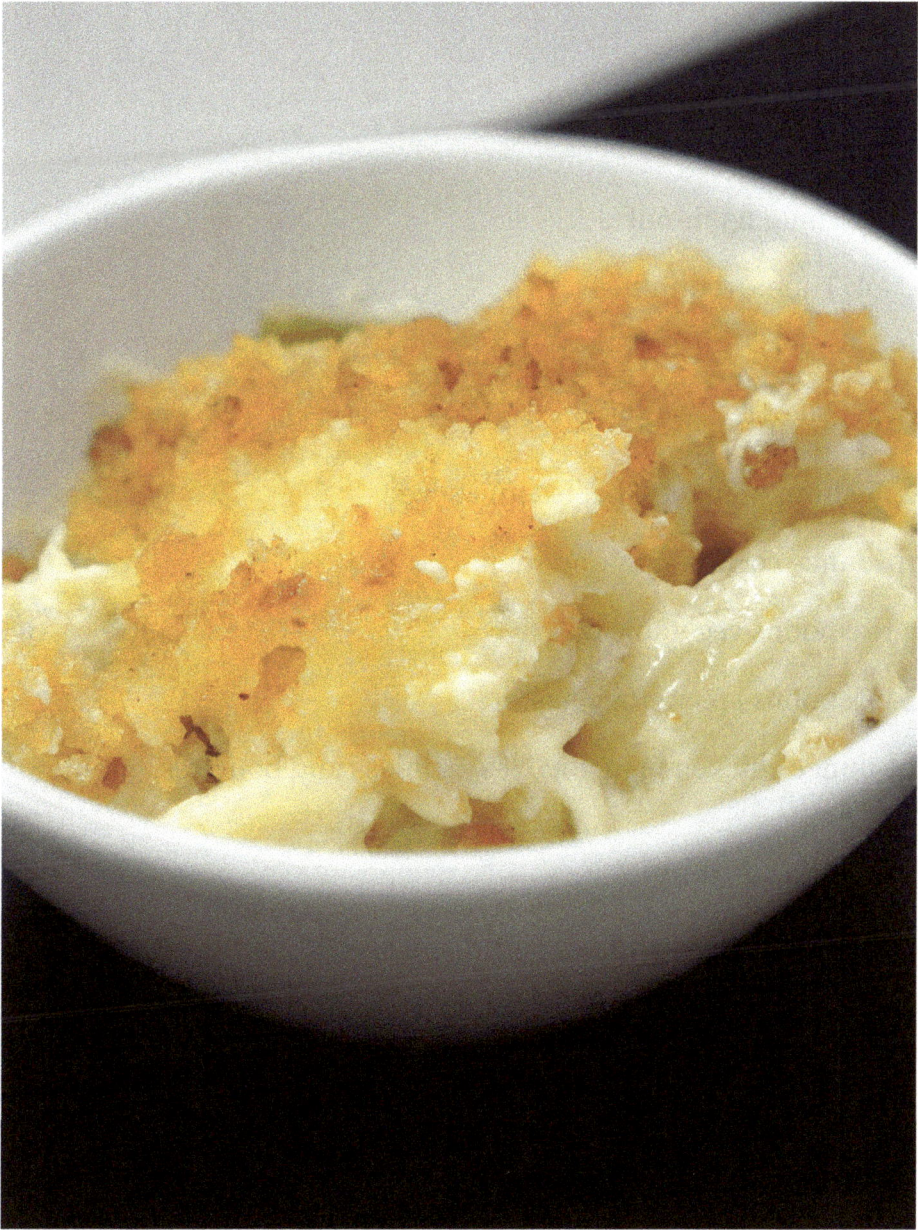

Epic Mango Chicken

Serving: 4

Prep Time: 25 minutes

Cook Time: 10 minutes

Ingredients:

2 medium mangoes, peeled and sliced

10-ounce coconut almond milk

4 teaspoons vegetable oil

4 teaspoons spicy curry paste

14-ounce chicken breast halves, skinless and boneless, cut in cubes

4 medium shallots

1 large English cucumber, sliced and seeded

How To:

1.   Slice half the mangoes and add the halves to a bowl.

2.   Add mangoes and coconut almond milk to a blender and blend until you've got a smooth puree.

3.	Keep the mixture on the side.

4.	Take a large-sized pot and place it over medium heat, add oil and permit the oil to heat up.

5.	Add curry paste and cook for 1 minute until you've got a pleasant fragrance, add shallots and chicken to the pot and cook for five minutes.

6.	Pour mango puree in to the combination and permit it to heat up.

7.	Serve the cooked chicken with mango puree and cucumbers.

8.	Enjoy!

Nutrition (Per Serving)

Calories: 398

Fat: 20g

Carbohydrates: 32g

Protein: 26g

Chicken and Cabbage Platter

Serving: 2

Prep Time: 9 minutes

Cook Time: 14 minutes

Ingredients:

½ cup sliced onion

1 tablespoon sesame garlic-flavored oil 2cups shredded Bok-Choy 1/2 cups fresh bean sprouts

1 1/2 stalks celery, chopped

1 ½ teaspoons minced garlic

1/2 teaspoon stevia

1/2 cup chicken broth

1 tablespoon coconut aminos

1/2 tablespoon freshly minced ginger

1/2 teaspoon arrowroot

2 boneless chicken breasts, cooked and sliced thinly

How To:

1.   Shred the cabbage with a knife.

2.   Slice onion and increase your platter alongside the rotisserie chicken.

3.   Add a dollop of mayonnaise on top and drizzle vegetable oil over the cabbage.

4.   Season with sunflower seeds and pepper consistent with your taste.

5.   Enjoy!

Nutrition (Per Serving)

Calories: 368

Fat: 18g

Net Carbohydrates: 8g

Protein: 42g

Fiber: 3g

Carbohydrates: 11g

Hearty Chicken Liver Stew

Serving: 2

Prep Time: 10 minutes

Cook Time: Nil

Ingredients:

10 ounces chicken livers

1-ounce onion, chopped

2 ounces sour cream

1 tablespoon olive oil

Sunflower seeds to taste

How To:

1. Take a pan and place it over medium heat.

2. Add oil and let it heat up.

3. Add onions and fry until just browned.

4. Add livers and season with sunflower seeds.

5. Cook until livers are half cooked.

6. Transfer the combination to a stew pot.

7.   Add soured cream and cook for 20 minutes.

8.   Serve and enjoy!

Nutrition (Per Serving)

Calories: 146

Fat: 9g

Carbohydrates: 2g

Protein: 15g

Chicken Quesadilla

Serving: 2

Prep Time: 10 minutes

Cook Time: 35 minutes

Ingredients:

¼ cup ranch dressing

½ cup cheddar cheese, shredded

20 slices bacon, center-cut

2 cups grilled chicken, sliced

How To:

1.   Re-heat your oven to 400 degrees F.

2.   Line baking sheet using parchment paper.

3.   Weave bacon into two rectangles and bake for half-hour.

4.   Lay grilled chicken over bacon square, drizzling ranch dressing on top.

5.   Sprinkle cheddar and top with another bacon square.

6. Bake for five minutes more.

7. Slice and serve.

8. Enjoy!

Nutrition (Per Serving)

Calories: 619

Fat: 35g

Carbohydrates: 2g

Protein: 79g

Zucchini Beef Sauté with

Coriander Greens

Serving: 4

Prep Time: 10 minutes

Cook Time: 10 minutes

Ingredients:

10 ounces beef, sliced into 1-2-inch strips

1 zucchini, cut into 2-inch strips

¼ cup parsley, chopped

3 garlic cloves, minced

2 tablespoons tamari sauce

4 tablespoons avocado oil

How To:

1.   Add 2 tablespoons avocado oil during a frypan over high heat.

2.   Place strips of beef and brown for a couple of minutes on high heat.

3.   Once the meat is brown, add zucchini strips and sauté until tender.

4.   Once tender, add tamari sauce, garlic, parsley and allow them to sit for a couple of minutes more.

5.   Serve immediately and enjoy!

Nutrition (Per Serving)

Calories: 500

Fat: 40g

Carbohydrates: 5g

Protein: 31g

Hearty Lemon and Pepper Chicken

Serving: 4

Prep Time: 5 minutes

Cook Time: 15

Ingredients:

2 teaspoons olive oil

1 ¼ pounds skinless chicken cutlets

2 whole eggs

¼ cup panko crumbs

1 tablespoon lemon pepper

Sunflower seeds and pepper to taste

3 cups green beans

¼ cup parmesan cheese

¼ teaspoon garlic powder

How To:

1.   Pre-heat your oven to 425 degrees F.

2. Take a bowl and stir in seasoning, parmesan, lemon pepper, garlic powder, panko.

3. Whisk eggs in another bowl.

4. Coat cutlets in eggs and press into panko mix.

5. Transfer coated chicken to a parchment lined baking sheet.

6. Toss the beans in oil, pepper, add sunflower seeds, and lay them on the side of the baking sheet.

7. Bake for quarter-hour.

8. Enjoy!

Nutrition (Per Serving)

Calorie: 299

Fat: 10g

Carbohydrates: 10g

Protein: 43g

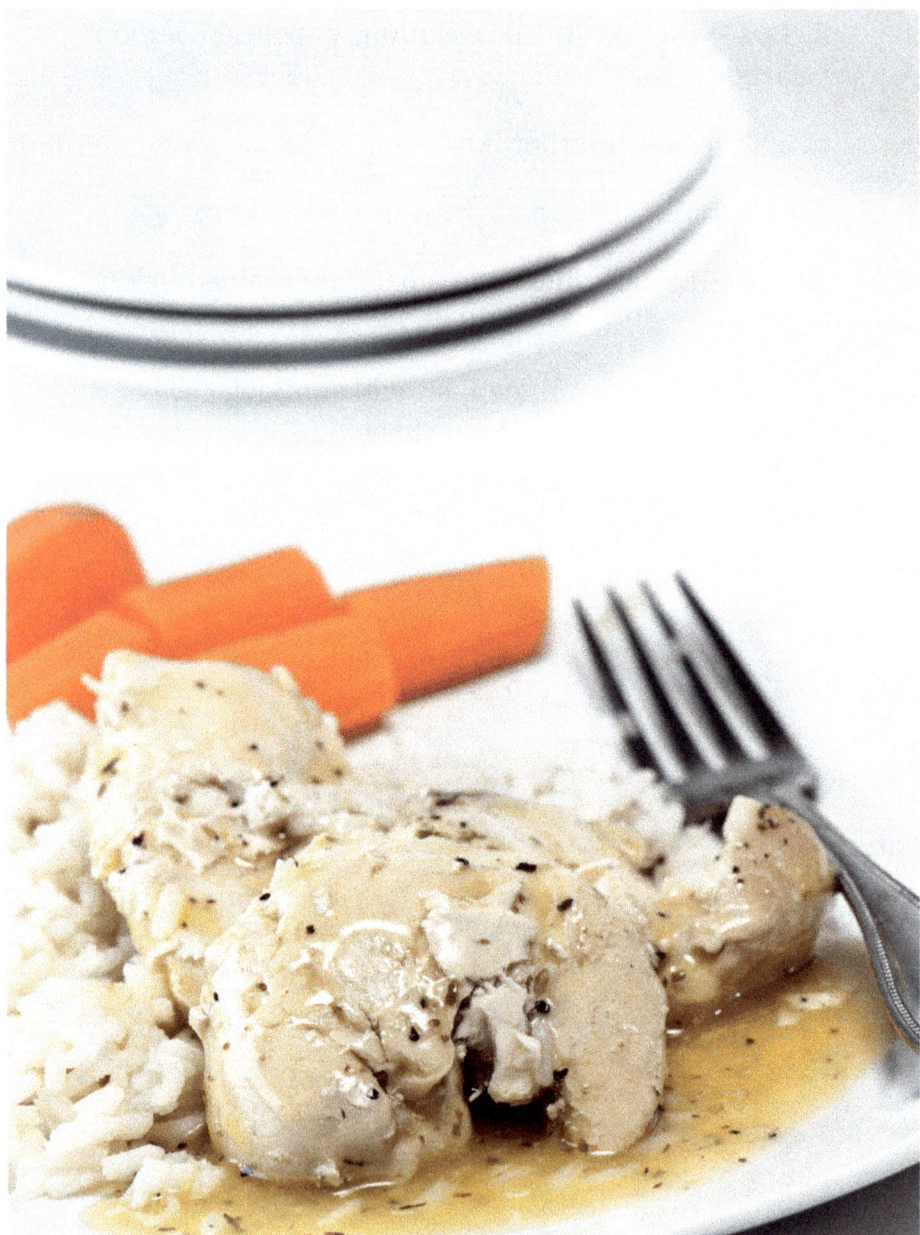

Walnuts and Asparagus Delight

Serving: 4

Prep Time: 5 minutes

Cook Time: 5 minutes

Ingredients:

1 ½ tablespoons olive oil

¾ pound asparagus, trimmed

¼ cup walnuts, chopped

Sunflower seeds and pepper to taste

How To:

1.   Place a skillet over medium heat add vegetable oil and let it heat up.

2.   Add asparagus, sauté for five minutes until browned.

3.   Season with sunflower seeds and pepper.

4.   Remove heat.

5.   Add walnuts and toss.

6.   Serve warm!

Nutrition (Per Serving)

Calories: 124

Fat: 12g

Carbohydrates: 2g

Protein: 3g

Healthy Carrot Chips

Serving: 4

Prep Time: 10 minutes

Cook Time: 10 minutes

Ingredients:

3 cups carrots, sliced paper-thin rounds

2 tablespoons olive oil

2 teaspoons ground cumin

½ teaspoon smoked paprika Pinch of sunflower seeds

How To:

1.   Pre-heat your oven to 400 degrees F.

2.   Slice carrot into thin shaped coins employing a peeler.

3.   Place slices during a bowl and toss with oil and spices.

4.   Lay out the slices on a parchment paper, lined baking sheet during a single layer.

5.   Sprinkle sunflower seeds.

6.   Transfer to oven and bake for 8-10 minutes.

7.   Remove and serve.

Enjoy!

Nutrition (Per Serving)

Calories: 434

Fat: 35g

Carbohydrates: 31g

Protein: 2g

Garden Vegetable and Herb Soup

Total Time

Prep: 20 min. Cook: 30 min.

Makes

8 servings (2 quarts)

Ingredients:

2 tablespoons olive oil

2 medium onions, hacked

2 huge carrots, cut

1 pound red potatoes (around 3 medium), cubed

2 cups of water

1 can (14-1/2 ounces) diced tomatoes in sauce

1-1/2 cups vegetable soup

1-1/2 teaspoons garlic powder

1 teaspoon dried basil

1/2 teaspoon salt

1/2 teaspoon paprika

1/4 teaspoon dill weed

1/4 teaspoon pepper

1 medium yellow summer squash, split and cut

1 medium zucchini, split and cut

Directions:

1.   In a huge pan, heat oil over medium warmth. Include onions and carrots; cook and mix until onions are delicate, 4-6 minutes. Include potatoes and cook 2 minutes. Mix in water, tomatoes, juices, and seasonings. Heat to the point of boiling. Diminish heat; stew, revealed, until potatoes and carrots are delicate, 9 minutes.

2.   Include yellow squash and zucchini; cook until vegetables are delicate, 9 minutes longer. Serve or, whenever wanted, puree blend in clusters, including extra stock until wanted consistency is accomplished.

Salad Chard and White Bean Pasta

Total Time

Prep: 20 min. Cook: 20 min.

Makes

8 servings

Ingredients:

1 bundle (12 ounces) uncooked entire wheat or darker rice penne pasta

2 tablespoons olive oil

4 cups cut leeks (a white bit as it were)

1 cup cut sweet onion

4 garlic cloves, cut

1 tablespoon minced crisp savvy or 1 teaspoon scoured sage

1 enormous sweet potato, stripped and cut into 1/2-inch solid shapes

1 medium bundle Swiss chard (around 1 pound), cut into 1-inch cuts

1 can (15-1/2 ounces) extraordinary northern beans, flushed and depleted

3/4 teaspoon salt

1/4 teaspoon bean stew powder

1/4 teaspoon squashed red pepper drops 1/8 teaspoon ground nutmeg 1/8 teaspoon pepper

1/3 cup finely slashed crisp basil

1 tablespoon balsamic vinegar

2 cups marinara sauce, warmed

Directions:

1.   Cook pasta as indicated by bundle headings. Channel, holding 3/4 cup pasta water.

2.   In a 6-qt. stockpot, heat oil over medium warmth; saute leeks and onion until delicate, 5-7 minutes. Include garlic and sage; cook and mix 2 minutes.

3.   Include potato and chard; cook, secured, over medium-low warmth 5 minutes. Mix in beans, seasonings and held pasta water; cook, secured, until potato and chard are delicate, around 5 minutes.

4.   Include pasta, basil, and vinegar; hurl and warmth through. Present with sauce.

Cauliflower with Roasted Almond and Pepper Dip

Total Time

Prep: 40 min. Bake: 35 min.

Makes

10 servings (2-1/4 cups dip)

Ingredients:

10 cups water

1 cup olive oil, isolated

3/4 cup sherry or red wine vinegar, isolated

3 tablespoons salt

1 cove leaf

1 tablespoon squashed red pepper drops

1 enormous head cauliflower

1/2 cup entire almonds, toasted

1/2 cup delicate entire wheat or white bread morsels, toasted 1/2 cup fire-simmered squashed tomatoes

1 container (8 ounces) broiled sweet red peppers, depleted

2 tablespoons minced new parsley

2 garlic cloves

1 teaspoon sweet paprika

1/2 teaspoon salt

1/4 teaspoon newly ground pepper

Directions:

1.　　In a 6-qt. stockpot, bring water, 1/2 cup oil, 1/2 cup sherry, salt, sound leaf, and pepper pieces to a bubble. Include cauliflower. Diminish heat; stew, revealed, until a blade effectively embeds into focus, 15-20 minutes, turning part of the way through cooking. Evacuate with an opened spoon; channel well on paper towels.

2.　　Preheat broiler to 450°. Spot cauliflower on a lubed wire rack in a 15x10x1-in. heating dish. Prepare on a lower broiler rack until dim brilliant, 39 minutes.

3.　　In the meantime, place almonds, bread morsels, tomatoes, cooked peppers, parsley, garlic, paprika, salt, and pepper in a nourishment processor; beat until finely cleaved. Include remaining sherry; process until mixed. Keep preparing while step by step including remaining oil in a constant flow. Present with cauliflower.

Spicy Grilled Broccoli

Total Time

Prep: 20 min. + standing Grill: 10 min.

Makes

6 servings

Ingredients:

2 packs broccoli

MARINADE:

1/2 cup olive oil

1/4 cup juice vinegar

1 teaspoon onion powder

1 teaspoon garlic powder

1 teaspoon smoked paprika

1/2 teaspoon salt

1/2 teaspoon squashed red pepper pieces 1/4 teaspoon pepper

Direction:

1.   Cut every broccoli pack into 6 pieces. In a 6-qt. stockpot, place a steamer container more than 1 in. of water. Spot broccoli in bushel. Heat water to the point of boiling. Decrease warmth to keep up a stew; steam, secured, 4-6 minutes or until fresh delicate.

2.   In an enormous bowl, whisk marinade fixings until mixed. Include broccoli; delicately hurl to cover. Let stand, secured, 15 minutes.

3.   Channel broccoli, saving marinade. Flame broil broccoli, secured, over medium warmth or cook 4 in. from heat 6-8 minutes or until broccoli is delicate, turning once. Whenever wanted, present withheld marinade.

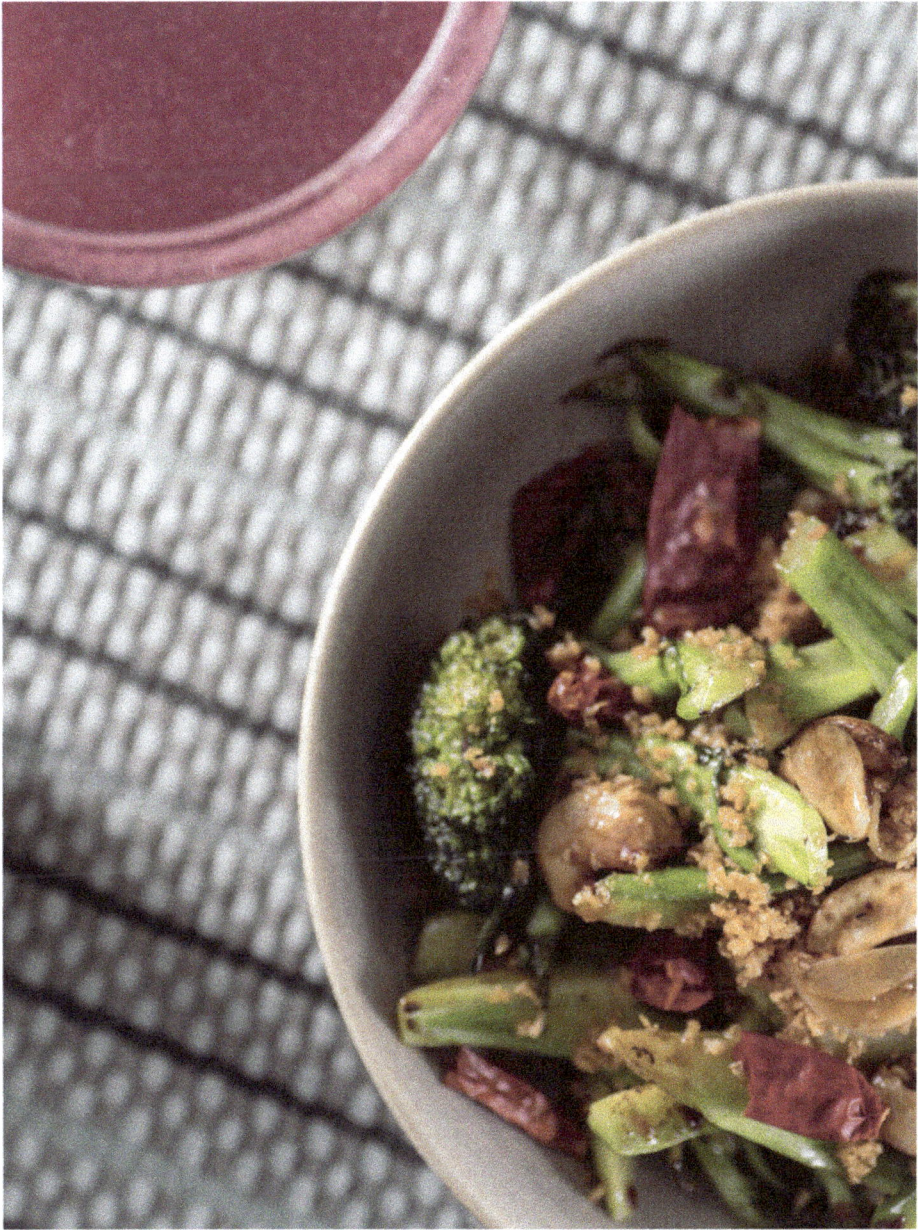

Super-easy Chicken Noodle Soup

SmartPoints value: Green plan - 3SP, Blue plan - 2SP, Purple plan - 2SP

Total Time: 32 min, Prep time: 12 min, Cooking time: 20 min, Serves: 8

Nutritional value: Calories - 351.3, Carbs - 37.3g, Fat - 4.5g, Protein - 39.7g

In this recipe, I will make it easy for you to prepare a hearty soup for the whole family, all with just one pot. A big cup of 1 1/2 portion has only two SmartPoints value, so it's perfect for lunch, either to take to work or for your child's lunchbox, too.

Unlike other recipes like it, this one will be ready in just 32 minutes, not hours!

Now, pick up some ZeroPoint chicken breasts, frozen vegetables, a box of pasta, chicken broth, and a few more bits and pieces, and let's get you started on this family delight.

Ingredients

Black pepper - ¼ tsp

Chicken breast(s) (cooked) - 6 oz, chopped (skinless, boneless)

Salted butter - 2 tsp

Onion(s) (uncooked)- 1 large, well chopped

Table salt - 1½ tsp, divided

Chicken broth (reduced-sodium) - 64 oz

Pasta (uncooked) - 4 oz, small shape such as ditalini (about 1 cup)

Mixed vegetables (frozen) - 10 oz, such as peas, green beans, and carrots

Tomatoes (canned) - 15 oz, petite cut, rinsed and drained

Parmesan cheese (grated) - 1 Tbsp

Lemon juice (fresh) - 2 tsp

Fresh chives - ¼ cup(s), chopped (optional)

Instructions

1.   Melt two teaspoons of butter in a large stockpot over medium-low heat.

2.   Add well-chopped onion and 1/2 teaspoon of salt, then cook, often stirring, until the onion is soft and translucent; about 10 minutes.

3.   Add the broth in the chicken and increase the heat to high, then bring it to a boil.

4.   Put in the pasta, frozen vegetables, and tomatoes, then cook until pasta is soft; about 7 minutes.

5.   Stir in the chicken, lemon juice, cheese, remaining one teaspoon of salt, black pepper, and chives, then cook one more minute to heat through.

Hearty Ginger Soup

Serving: 4

Prep Time: 5 minutes

Cook Time: 5 minutes

Ingredients:

3 cups coconut almond milk

2 cups water

½ pound boneless chicken breast halves, cut into chunks 3 tablespoons fresh ginger root, minced 2 tablespoons fish sauce

¼ cup fresh lime juice

2 tablespoons green onions, sliced

1 tablespoon fresh cilantro, chopped

How To:

1.   Take a saucepan and add coconut almond milk and water.

2.   Bring the mixture to a boil and add the chicken strips.

3.   Reduce the warmth to medium and simmer for 3 minutes.

4. Stir within the ginger, juice , and fish sauce.

5. Sprinkle a couple of green onions and cilantro.

6. Serve!

Nutrition (Per Serving)

Calories: 415

Fat: 39g

Carbohydrates: 8g

Protein: 14g

Tasty Tofu and Mushroom Soup

Serving: 8

Prep Time: 10 minutes

Cook Time: 10 minutes

Ingredients:

3 cups prepared dashi stock

¼ cup shiitake mushrooms, sliced

1 tablespoon miso paste

1 tablespoon coconut aminos

1/8 cup cubed soft tofu

1 green onion, diced

How To:

1.   Take a saucepan and add stock, bring back a boil.

2.   Add mushrooms, cook for 4 minutes.

3.   Take a bowl and add coconut aminos, miso paste and blend well.

4.   Pour the mixture into stock and let it cook for six minutes on simmer.

5.   Add diced green onions and enjoy!

Nutrition (Per Serving)

Calories: 100

Fat: 4g

Carbohydrates: 5g

Protein: 11

Ingenious Eggplant Soup

Serving: 8

Prep Time: 20 minutes

Cook Time: 15 minutes

Ingredients:

1 large eggplant, washed and cubed

1 tomato, seeded and chopped

1 small onion, diced

2 tablespoons parsley, chopped

2 tablespoons extra virgin olive oil

2 tablespoons distilled white vinegar

½ cup parmesan cheese, crumbled Sunflower seeds as needed

How To:

1.   Pre-heat your outdoor grill to medium-high.

2.   Pierce the eggplant a couple of times employing a knife/fork.

3.   Cook the eggplants on your grill for about quarter-hour

until they're charred.

4.   forgot and permit them to chill .

5.   Remove the skin from the eggplant and dice the pulp.

6.   Transfer the pulp to a bowl and add parsley, onion, tomato, olive oil, feta cheese and vinegar.

7.   Mix well and chill for 1 hour.

8.   Season with sunflower seeds and enjoy!

Nutrition (Per Serving)

Calories: 99

Fat: 7g

Carbohydrates: 7g

Protein:3.4g

Loving Cauliflower Soup

Serving: 6

Prep Time: 10 minutes

Cook Time: 10 minutes

Ingredients:

4 cups vegetable stock

1-pound cauliflower, trimmed and chopped

7 ounces Kite ricotta/cashew cheese

4 ounces almond butter

Sunflower seeds and pepper to taste

How To:

1.   Take a skillet and place it over medium heat.

2.   Add almond butter and melt.

3.   Add cauliflower and sauté for two minutes.

4.   Add stock and convey mix to a boil.

5.   Cook until cauliflower is hard .

6.   Stir in cheese, sunflower seeds and pepper.

7.   Puree the combination using an immersion blender.

8.   Serve and enjoy!

Nutrition (Per Serving)

Calories: 143

Fat: 16g

Carbohydrates: 6g

Protein: 3.4g

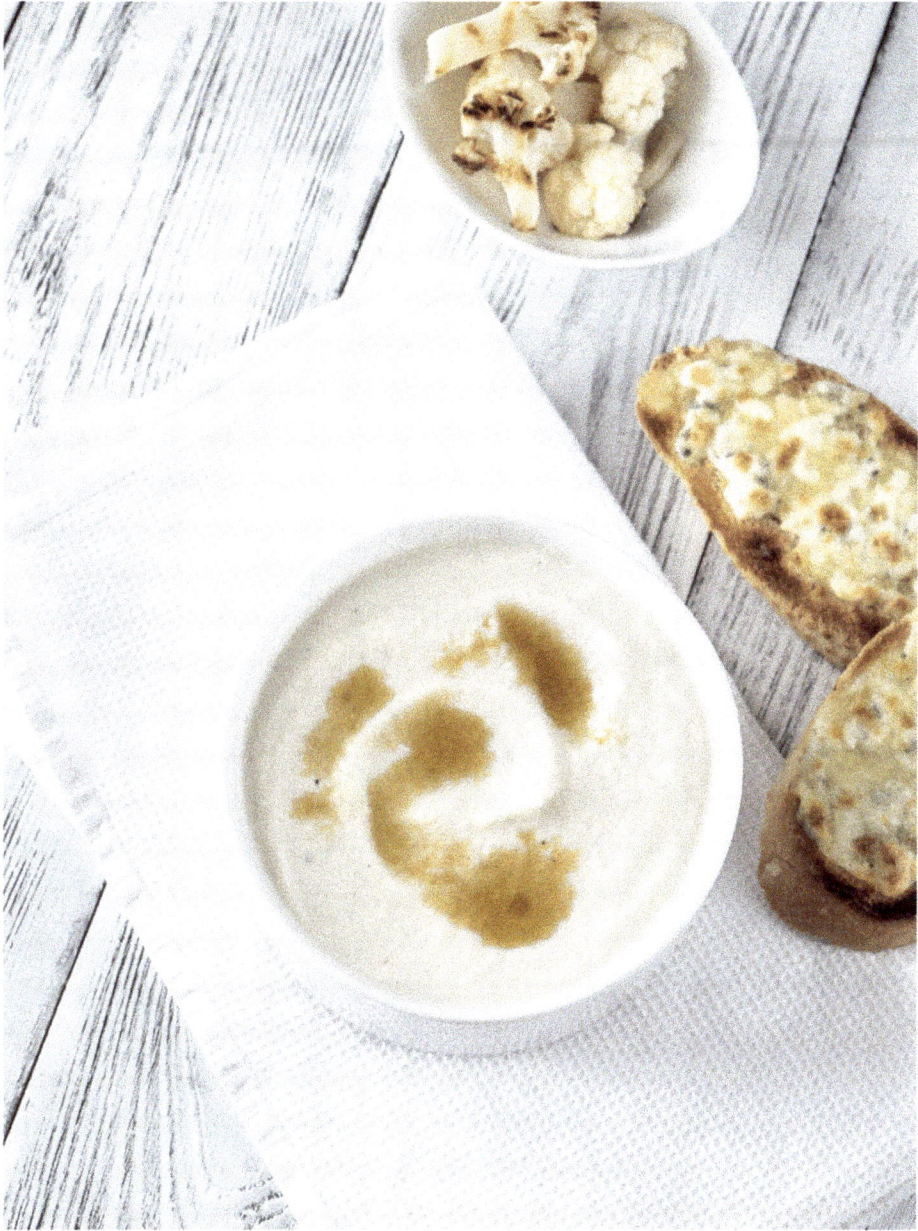

www.ingramcontent.com/pod-product-compliance
Lightning Source LLC
Chambersburg PA
CBHW050745030426
42336CB00012B/1667